# HOMEMADE NATURAL HERBAL REMEDIES FOR SCLERODERMA

By Smith J. Offor

# Table of Contents

# Introduction

**11 home remedies and prevention advice for scleroderma**

**What Is Sclerodermia?**

A group of autoimmune diseases known as scleroderma cause the skin and connective tissue in your body to tighten and harden. It is a chronic condition with a propensity to worsen over time. Anti-nuclear antibodies, which cause immunological problems because scleroderma is an autoimmune disease, are one of the symptoms . The most notable ones are anti-topoisomerase antibodies, anti-RNA polymerase III antibodies, and anti-centromere antibodies.

Systemic sclerosis and crest syndrome are other names for scleroderma. It is regarded as a rheumatic condition.

With an incidence of 3 cases per 100,000 people per year, localized scleroderma primarily affects women.

An immune system issue that results in increased collagen production is the cause of scleroderma. The protein known as collagen is what holds your skin, muscles, tendons, and bones together. Your tissues become thicker and scarred as a result of excessive collagen production. Scleroderma ranges in severity from mild to possibly fatal.

Scleroderma is typically divided into two types:

- restricted scleroderma

- Systemic sclerosis

The various forms of scleroderma and the associated symptoms are listed below.

# SCLERODERMA TYPES AND SYMPTOMS

## Scleroderma that is localized

Localized scleroderma primarily impacts the skin, though it can also have an effect on your muscles and bones. The internal organs are unaffected and it is the mildest type of scleroderma. It is further divided into two types: linear scleroderma and morphea.

Oval-shaped light or dark patches on your skin are one of the signs of morphea scleroderma.

Bands or streaks of hardened skin may form on the limbs in people with linear scleroderma. Joint pain is typically caused by how it affects the muscles and bones.

**Scleroderma systemica**
The entire body is impacted by systemic scleroderma, including the blood and internal organs like the kidneys, esophagus, lungs, and heart. It is connected to fibrosis in various organs. Limited cutaneous systemic sclerosis syndrome (CREST) and diffuse cutaneous systemic sclerosis are its two primary subtypes. Additionally, they are referred to as diffuse and limited scleroderma. The condition's least serious form is called limited cutaneous systemic sclerosis syndrome (CREST). Typically, the skin on your hands, face, feet, lower arms, and legs is affected. The acronym CREST,

which stands for: is formed by the symptoms of this syndrome, which is why it is also known as CREST syndrome.

The formation of calcium deposits in tissues and beneath the skin is known as calcinosis.

## Raynaud's syndrome

- E - Esophageal conditions like GERD.
- Sclerodactyly is the formation of thick skin on the fingers.
- Blood vessel enlargement that appears as red spots is known as telangiectasia (T).

The thickening of the skin on your hands and wrists is a sign of diffuse systemic sclerosis. It may also have an impact on your internal organs. Weakness, fatigue, weight loss, difficulty breathing, and difficulty swallowing are symptoms that affected people frequently experience.

Scleroderma signs and symptoms are mainly:

- stiffness, tightness, and puffiness in your fingers and hands as a result of emotional stress or cold sensitivity.
- Intensification in the feet.
- calcium buildup.
- digital ulcers may result from the narrowing of blood vessels in the hands and feet (Raynaud's disease).
- difficulties with the esophagus
- skin on the fingers has thickened
- red spots start to appear on the hands and face

This condition's precise cause is still unknown. Nevertheless, given that it is an autoimmune condition, issues with your immune system's performance may be the main contributing factor. The following list includes additional risk factors or causes for scleroderma.

# 16 HOME TREATMENTS FOR SWOLLEN FT SYMPTOMS, AND SOLUTIONS

**Risk factors and their causes.**
Scleroderma risk factors include diabetes.

The overproduction of collagen, a protein that serves as the foundation of connective tissues, is thought to be one of the primary causes of scleroderma. The affected tissues may become thicker and eventually scar.

Genes may be another factor contributing to the onset of scleroderma. It hasn't yet been confirmed, though.

People with scleroderma frequently have autoimmune disease histories in their families, which adds another risk factor that could be influencing the development of the disease.

Your risk of developing scleroderma may also be affected by:

**Age:** Scleroderma is more likely to develop in people between the ages of 30 and 50.

**Gender** – Women are more likely to contract this illness.

Scleroderma is more likely to develop if you have medical conditions like diabetes.

exposure to environmental elements like silica dust and specific chemicals like vinyl chloride.

Your risk is also increased by drugs like bleomycin and carbidopa.

**Protip icon a fast tip**
Scleroderma may result in functional limitations, particularly in the hands and

mouth, which may affect how food is consumed.

Since it manifests gradually and in a variety of ways, scleroderma is very challenging to diagnose. Consequently, your doctor may perform the following tests to make a diagnosis.

## Diagnosis

To diagnose scleroderma, your doctor may perform a physical examination in addition to some other tests. These examinations consist of:.

checking the skin under a microscope for any alterations.

**Biopsy**

Tests on the blood to determine the presence of various antibodies.

Before determining the cause of your condition, your doctor may also look for symptoms of skin thickening, shortness of breath, GERD, and calcium deposition.

Your doctor may advise any of the following therapies once you have been definitively diagnosed with scleroderma.

**Techniques for treatment**

There are several medical remedies for scleroderma.

- Blood pressure medications to help treat Raynaud's phenomenon or disease, which arises from scleroderma, and to widen your blood vessels

- Immunosuppressive drugs to reduce immune system activity
- Physical therapy can help you feel better, move better, and be stronger
- To enhance the look and condition of your skin, consider laser surgery or UV light therapy

Here are a few all-natural remedies for treating this condition.

## Natural Scleroderma Management Techniques

- Calcium D.
- oil essentials.
- "Gotu Kola.".
- Turmeric.
- Onion.

- Lemon.

- A gram of flour

- fatty fish

- Ginger

- The cottage cheese

# Home Treatments for the Symptoms Of Scleroderma

1. The vitamin D.

## What is required of you

You can either eat foods like fatty fish, cheese, and egg yolks that are high in vitamin D, or you can take supplements.

Before ingesting supplements, seek medical advice.

## How Often Should You Perform This

- Engage in this routinely.

## Why It Works

The symptoms of scleroderma can be effectively managed with vitamin D due to its immunomodulatory, antifibrotic, and cardioprotective effects.

The majority of sclerodermic people also lack enough vitamin D, indicating the necessity of supplementation.

### 2. Scented oils

Symptoms of scleroderma are managed by a blend of essential oils. Save.

## a. Oil of peppermint

It Is Required.

Peppermint oil, 6 drops.

Coconut oil (or another carrier oil) in the amount of one teaspoon.

## What is required of you.

- A teaspoon of coconut oil should have six drops of peppermint oil added to it.
- Apply it to the affected area after thoroughly mixing.
- It can be left on all night or for 30 minutes.
- Wash it off with water

# How Often Should You Perform This?

This can be done once or twice every day.

## What Makes This Work

Because menthol is present, peppermint oil has a calming and anti-inflammatory effect on inflamed and swollen skin. Additionally, it can aid in reducing pain symptoms.

### b. Oil of Lavender

You'll require.

- Lavender oil, six drops.
- 1 teaspoon of carrier oil—coconut or another—is required.

## You must do this

- A teaspoon of any carrier oil should contain six drops of lavender oil.
- Apply it to the skin that is affected after thoroughly mixing.
- Leave it on overnight if possible, or for 20 to 30 minutes
- Wash it off with water

## How Often Should You Perform This

This can be done once or twice every day.

## Why It Functions

It is not surprising that lavender oil is effective in treating the pain and inflammation associated with scleroderma because of its anti-inflammatory and analgesic properties. Also, it lowers stress levels.

## 3. Goto Kola

## You'll Need:

- dried gotu kola, about a half-teaspoon
- hot water in one glass

## What is required of you

- To a cup of hot water, add half a teaspoon of dried gotu kola
- Strain after steeping for 5 to 7 minutes
- Take some of the tea

## How Frequently You Should Do This

- 1-3 times a day, sip gotu kola tea.

## Why It Works

The medicinal herb centella asiatica, also known as gotu kola, is well known for promoting the health of your blood vessels and stabilizing connective tissues. Inflammation and stress symptoms can both be reduced by it.

## 4. Turmeric

You'll Need.

- Powdered turmeric, 1 teaspoon
- 1 glass of hot water or milk

**You must do this.**

- In a glass of hot milk or water, stir one teaspoon of turmeric powder
- Combine thoroughly
- ingest the mixture
- The affected skin can also be covered in a paste made of turmeric and water, which you should leave on for a few minutes

## When You Should Repeat This

- This is something you could do once every day.

## How Come This Works

Curcumin is plentiful in turmeric. The overproduction of collagen and subsequent development of scleroderma were observed to be suppressed by curcumin supplementation.

## 5. Onion

It Is Required

- a little onion.

## What is required of you

- Make two halves of a small onion
- Gently massage the afflicted area with the onion half
- For 20 to 30 minutes, let the skin absorb the onion extract
- Clean it with water

## How Frequently You Should Do This

Perform this once or twice each day.

## Why It Works

Cepaene and thiosulfinates, which have anti-inflammatory properties, are abundant in onions.

This helps to reduce the signs of swelling and inflammation.

## 6. Lemon

Scleroderma can be treated with lemon and honey.

It Is Required

- 1 lemon.
- 1 spoonful of honey.

## What You Must Do

- The lemon's juice should be extracted
- A teaspoon of honey should be added
- Put some of the mixture on the skin that is harmed
- It should be left on for 20 minutes
- Clean it with water

## How Frequently You Must Do This

This has to be done once every day.

## How Come This Works

Applying lemon juice topically helps to soften the thickened skin and reduces swelling and inflammation.

## 7. Flour in grams

In order to:

- Gram flour, 2 teaspoons
- Water, as needed

## What You Must Do

To make a paste, combine two teaspoons of gram flour with a little water.

In the affected area, evenly distribute the paste, and then leave it on for at least 20 minutes.

With some water, remove it.

Additionally, you can use this mixture as a soap substitute that is natural.

How Frequently You Must Do This.

Use this on your skin at least once per day.

## What Makes This Work

Skin that has thickened and become rough can benefit from the use of gram flour. It also aids in restoring the texture of your skin.

## 8. Oil from fish (Omega 3)

In order to:

omega-3 fish oil in doses of 250–500 mg.

You must do this:

- Take between 250 and 500 mg of fish oil every day.
- You can eat fatty fish like tuna, salmon, and mackerel.
- You could also take fish oil supplements.

- How Frequently You Must Do This

- Include fish oil in your diet on a regular basis

## Why It Functions

Omega-3 fatty acids, which are abundant in fish oil, are beneficial for lowering swelling and inflammation in the body. One of the symptoms of scleroderma, Raynaud's disease, can be avoided by consuming fish oil (11).

## 9. Ginger

In order to

- Ginger that is between one and two inches long.

- one cup of hot water.

**You must do this**

- One to two inches of ginger should be added to a cup of hot water.
- After 5 to 10 minutes of steeping, strain.
- Consume the hot tea.

**How Often Should You Perform This**

You can have two to three daily cups of ginger tea.

**Why It Functions**

Because ginger has potent anti-inflammatory and antioxidant properties, it can help you manage the signs and symptoms of scleroderma by preventing the production of prostaglandins in your body that cause pain.

## 10.    Panela, or cottage cheese

It Is Required:

Cottage cheese, 2 portions.

## what is required of you.

- Add cottage cheese to your favorite dishes or salads
- When You Should Repeat This
- Cottage cheese is a food that you can have once a day

## How Come This Works.

Sulfur is found in abundance in cottage cheese, which makes it easier for your cells to absorb oil and other nutrients. This gives you more energy and makes it easier for you to manage your scleroderma.

A natural alternative to these treatments for managing scleroderma symptoms is to make dietary changes.

For those who are battling sclerode, the diet listed below was created.

- Cottage cheese has thirteen health benefits, and it is also nutritious.
- diet for scleroderma.
- Scleroderma management with turmeric, ginger, and cinnamon.
- Scleroderma patients are typically advised to eat small meals every three to four hours
- Increase your intake of the following anti-inflammatory and antioxidant herbs and spices

## Foods To Consume

- Basil.
- Rosemary
- Oregano
- Cinnamon
- Paprika
- Ginger
- Cayenne
- Turmeric

Try to cut back on the foods listed below in your diet:

- Sugars that are totally free.
- Alcohol
- Caffeine

if you have GERD symptoms, stay away from foods like:

- citrus fruit.
- Tomatoes.
- unhealthy food
- Garlic
- Onions
- spicy cuisine
- carbonated drinks

The advice in the following paragraphs may be useful if you're looking for additional symptom management strategies.

## Advice for Managing Scleroderma

- Eat frequently and in smaller portions

- One or two hours before going to bed, avoid eating

- Maintain proper skin moisture

- Save your fingers from harm

- Keep warm to prevent circulatory problems

- Engage in stretching exercises to reduce stiffness

- Stop smoking.

- Stay away from using drugs for fun.

- Get adequate rest and sleep.

- To control your anxiety and stress, try yoga

- Avoid eating junk or processed food

- Avoid using herbs that are known to stimulate your immune system, such as echinacea

The overproduction of collagen in scleroderma, a rare progressive autoimmune disorder, causes the skin to tighten and harden and may even cause organ damage. It is a connective tissue disease that can be localized or systemic, and depending on which it is, it may have different symptoms. Localized scleroderma is a relatively milder form of the disorder, and its most noticeable symptoms are dark or light-colored bands or patches of hardened skin. Swelling, red spots, thickened fingers, stiffness, and other symptoms of systemic scleroderma can be seen. Some natural remedies for this condition include vitamin D, essential oils, gram flour, fish oil, lemon, and turmeric. Some types of scleroderma may also require medical treatment methods in addition to these. When necessary, it's crucial to get emotional and psychological support and to adhere to the treatment regimen advised by your doctor.

## Treatments for Scleroderma naturally

Scleroderma is the medical term for a condition that causes the skin or connective tissues—the fibers that support your skin and internal organs—to harden and thicken.

**Scleroderma comes in two main varieties:** localized and systemic. Systemic scleroderma affects your blood vessels and internal organs, including your heart and lungs, in addition to your skin, unlike localized scleroderma, which only affects your skin.

## Natural Treatments for Scleroderma

The use of complementary therapies to treat scleroderma is not well supported by scientific research. However, those looking to manage this condition might find the following treatments helpful.

## The vitamin D

Low vitamin D levels are frequently present in systemic sclerosis, according to a 2016 study involving 51 patients. The authors came to the conclusion that low vitamin status appears to be associated with a more aggressive disease with multivisceral and severe organ involvement, especially of the heart and lungs.

To determine the right daily dosage of vitamin D (a nutrient thought to help regulate the immune system), if you are dealing with systemic scleroderma, speak with your doctor.

## Vitamin E

Using topical vitamin E gel to treat digital ulcers brought on by systemic scleroderma may speed up healing and lessen pain, according to a 2009 study involving 27 patients.

An antifibrotic effect of vitamin E may help to prevent the accumulation of extra tissue, according to prior research.

## Symptoms of scleroderma

Oval-shaped, thickened patches of skin with a white center and a purple border are the hallmarks of morphea, one type of localized scleroderma.

The other type of localized scleroderma, known as linear scleroderma, is distinguished by bands or streaks of hardened skin on the arms, legs, or forehead. Depending on the part of the body that is affected by systemic scleroderma, a person's symptoms can change.

The following signs and symptoms of scleroderma can also appear:

- Raynaud's Syndrome.

- Your face and hands have red spots on them.

- Your fingers have thick, taut skin.

## What Leads to It?

Scleroderma has an unidentified exact cause. To the contrary, it is believed that excessive collagen production in cells results from abnormal immune system activity, which in turn leads to the accumulation of connective tissue. It is referred to as an autoimmune disease, which is a disease of the immune system, for this reason

Your risk of developing scleroderma may increase due to certain factors. These comprise:

- exposure to silica dust and specific industrial solvents (like paint thinners).

- receiving bleomycin as part of a specific type of chemotherapy.

- African-Americans and some Native American tribes, such as the Choctaw Native Americans of Oklahoma, seem to be at a higher risk for developing scleroderma or its complications.

## Alternative Therapies

If you exhibit symptoms of scleroderma, you should see a doctor right away because this condition can cause serious complications that can be fatal (like irreparable damage to the heart, lungs, or kidneys).

Although there is currently no way to stop the overproduction of collagen and cure scleroderma, certain medical treatments can help manage symptoms and limit damage. Depending on the areas affected, the treatment may involve using medication, surgery, and/or physical therapy.

# SCLERODERMA TREATMENTS YOU CAN DO AT HOME

### What is sclerodermoderma?

A condition known as scleroderma causes the skin and connective tissues to harden and tighten. Scleroderma is divided into two main categories: systemic and localized. Scleroderma that is localized typically only affects the skin. Skin, supporting connective tissues, or significant organs are all affected by systemic scleroderma.

## At-home remedies

At-home remedies for scleroderma can help relieve symptoms in addition to standard medical care. Taking over-the-counter medications, protecting the skin and body from colds, exercising regularly, changing one's diet, and managing stress are some at-home treatment options.

## Medications available without a prescription

Various over-the-counter medications can be used to relieve specific symptoms of scleroderma:

- Gastroesophageal reflux disease can be alleviated by proton pump inhibitors like omeprazole.

- Stomach acid is lessened by H-2 blockers like ranitidine and famotidine.

- Heartburn can be relieved by antacids like calcium carbonate and magnesium hydroxide.

- Polyethylene glycol, docusate sodium, or bisacodyl are examples of medications that can ease constipation.

- Loperamide and bismuth subsalicylate are two examples of diarrhea treatments.

- Ibuprofen, naproxen sodium, and other NSAIDs can lessen pain and inflammation.

- Acetaminophen can aid in pain relief.

- Itching relief comes from topical medications like menthol or camphor.

- Treatments for dry mouth, such as carboxymethyl cellulose and hydroxyethyl cellulose, can aid in moisturizing the mouth.

- Artificial teardrops and other dry eye treatments aid in maintaining eye moisture

- Skin defense.

- Patches of dry, stiff skin are a symptom of scleroderma

**Reduce stiffness and dryness with the help of the following advice:**

- Regularly use lotion and apply sunscreen.

- Do not use harsh soaps or chemicals

- To keep the air moist, use a humidifier.

- Take a warm bath to lessen calcium deposits under the skin.

- protection from the cold.

- Reduced blood flow to the extremities in response to cold is a common scleroderma symptom known as Raynaud's disease. Raynaud's syndrome can be managed in a variety of ways:

- In order to allow for proper blood circulation to the extremities, keep the body warm in cold weather and stay away from tight clothing.

- In cold weather, dress in several warm layers.
- In chilly weather, wear mittens and a mask.
- physical exercise.
- Being active can maintain flexible joints and skin as well as improve circulation. You can try the following activities:.
- The heart's health and circulation are both aided by walking.
- Stretching the skin and joints through yoga is beneficial

## Diet

• Scleroderma, which frequently affects the digestive system, can cause weakness in the esophagus, stomach, and intestines.

45

The result could be a problem with food digestion.

• By implementing the following advice, the digestive systems can be lowered.

• You should stay away from foods that make you feel sick with heartburn or gastroesophageal reflux disease.

• Drink plenty of liquids. Water can also be used to soften food that is difficult to swallow.

• Eat frequently to help your body digest food more easily.

• By eating foods high in fiber, constipation can be lessened.

## Given dental care

For those who have scleroderma, dental care is essential because it raises the risk of tooth decay and cavities.

• Try to schedule at least one dental appointment every three months.

• Brush and floss your teeth thoroughly and on a regular basis.

• Use products to prevent dry mouth.


## Stress management.

• Stress can cause the body's inflammatory levels to increase.

• The suggestions listed below can help you feel less stressed.

• the exercise's pace.

47

Prioritizing tasks and identifying those that are particularly taxing can help you manage stress.

• creating a network of support.

• Helpful resources include upbeat people, actual support groups, and virtual (online) support groups.

## Sufficient relaxation

If you don't get enough sleep, your inflammation might get worse. Additionally, a bad night's sleep the night before frequently makes pain worse the next morning.

## Reversing Scleroderma Naturally

Actually a group of autoimmune diseases, scleroderma is characterized by hardened patches of connective tissue and skin. These patches, which can tighten up, can painfully restrict movement. Localized scleroderma typically only affects the skin, but in a small number of cases, it can also affect the muscles, joints, and bones. Scleroderma that is systemic is the more severe form. In addition to your digestive system and your kidneys, heart, and skin, it can also affect your lungs, heart, skin, muscles, and skin. 2 When it invades internal organs, it hardens and fibrousizes the tissues of those organs, reducing their functionality. Approximately 300,000 Americans suffer from scleroderma, a condition.

## The Common Treatment for Scleroderma.

Instead of offering actual treatments, traditional medicine uses harsh medications to mask your symptoms. Treatment is made more challenging by the fact that a lot of people with this condition experience depression due to the changes in their appearance. Even though they may not be signs of all types of scleroderma, facial changes, skin thickening, hair loss, and enlarged joints can make this autoimmune condition difficult to deal with. I want to reassure you that even though you might feel alone as a result of this condition, you are NOT alone and that you CAN take charge of your health and manage this condition.

This autoimmune disorder is brought on by the overproduction of collagen, a protein that is necessary for your connective tissue. This pertains to both your skin and digestive system.

**Symptoms of scleroderma.**

The tough, hardened, and occasionally discolored patches of skin are the most typical signs of localized scleroderma. Scleroderma known as morphea is characterized by waxy patches of skin that can change in size and even disappear. Linear scleroderma refers to bands or streaks of thick, hard skin on the arms, legs, or torso. Typically, only one side of the body experiences these bands. En coup de sabre5 (French for "sword wound") refers to linear streaks on the face that can resemble a cut from a knife or sword. Although they can affect adults as well, these types frequently affect children.

Women are four times more likely than men to develop systemic scleroderma, which primarily affects Caucasians in their 30s or 40s. Along with other symptoms, the most typical of which is Raynaud's Phenomenon, systemic scleroderma is characterized by the same thick skin patches as linear scleroderma. In Raynaud's Phenomenon, artery spasms lead to periods of decreased blood flow, typically in the fingers but occasionally in the toes, nose, lips, or ears. The affected areas briefly turn white or blue. The affected area turns red as blood starts to flow again, and most patients experience a burning, painful sensation.

## The Digestive System and Scleroderma.

The digestive system is the organ system that scleroderma patients most frequently experience damage to after the skin. Blood flow to the nerves that activate the bowel is decreased, which causes the intestines' muscles to gradually lose strength and tone and move slowly and erratically. Scleroderma patients may experience the typical IBS symptoms of bloating, constipation, and diarrhea. Additional signs include:.

• Calcium buildup beneath the skin.

- Joint pain.

- Weak muscles.

- Breathlessness.

- Dry cough.

- Swallowing issues.

- A reduction in weight.

- Reflux of acid8.


## Scleroderma's two types are diagnosed.

Rheumatologists or dermatologists are typically the ones who diagnose scleroderma. Because the condition mimics other disorders and there is no specific test for it, it is very difficult to diagnose. To determine whether you have the typical symptoms, your doctor will take a thorough medical history. Additionally, it's likely that he or she will request a blood test to check for specific autoantibodies linked to scleroderma. While MRIs can be used to evaluate soft tissue damage, other tests like CT scans and X-rays can help identify bone abnormalities.

## Scleroderma Conventional Treatments.

The underlying cause of scleroderma cannot be treated by conventional medicine. Instead of treating your body as a whole, a drug or treatment will typically be prescribed for each distinct symptom. For instance, medications like calcium channel blockers or medications known as

PDE-5 inhibitors, which widen constricted blood vessels and increase circulation, may be used to treat Raynaud's phenomenon. Immunosuppressive medications may be used to treat muscle pain and weakness, but these medications put you at risk for infections and other harmful side effects. Proton-pump inhibitors are another treatment for acid reflux that a doctor may recommend.

## How to Reverse Scleroderma Naturally.

Functional medicine seeks to treat the entire body while relieving symptoms in order to treat the underlying cause of a problem.

To lessen scleroderma's discomfort, do the following.

• Obtain adequate sleep.

• Sip a lot of purified water.

• Use soothing creams like shea butter or raw coconut oil.

• Protect and keep warm any skin that is exposed, especially your fingers and toes.

• Stretch your body gently to keep your skin and joints flexible. Yoga is a fantastic alternative.

• Moderate exercise will enhance blood circulation.

## The Natural Method to Treat Scleroderma.

You'll feel better after taking all of these steps. But identifying the underlying causes of your autoimmune condition and treating them is the key to effectively treating your scleroderma. There are alternatives to treating only the symptoms and resigning yourself to a lifetime of suffering from discomfort and embarrassment. I've created a four-pillar strategy that is very effective and can assist you in controlling the inflammation that is the main cause of most autoimmune diseases.

## Your Gut Will Heal

A healthy immune system depends on your gut being restored. Again, this is crucial for people with scleroderma whose digestive system tissues are compromised.

## Eliminate grains, legumes, and gluten

All of my patients have been advised to cut out gluten from their diets because it causes inflammation, which results in leaky gut. I also recommended eliminating all grains and legumes from the diets of people with autoimmune diseases, especially those with scleroderma whose digestive system tissues may be hardened. These foods contain lectins, a type of protein that acts as a natural pesticide on plants and can harm the lining of your gut. Several people find that avoiding dairy products, which are inflammatory foods, greatly improves their health.

## Subdue the toxins

You can control the toxins that are all around us by doing a number of things. Strong free-radical scavenger glutathione can enhance detoxification. This is crucial for anyone who has been exposed to toxic chemicals, especially silica, which has been linked to a higher incidence of systemic scleroderma. Scleroderma can also be effectively treated with hyperbaric therapy. Reduced inflammation and pain are the results of increased oxygen levels being injected into the bloodstream, which passes through the plasma.

## Reduce Stress and Heal Your Infections

There is simply no way to completely avoid stress. But one of the secrets to regaining control over your health is learning how to manage stress. It may take some trial and error to find the precise methods that are effective for you, but it is recommended that you try meditation, heart-math, yoga, walking, deep rhythmic breathing, journaling, and spending time with family and friends doing hobbies.

## Treatment

The excessive collagen production that is a defining feature of scleroderma cannot be reversed or treated. However, a number of treatments can help manage symptoms and avert complications.

## Medications

Depending on the symptoms of scleroderma, which can affect so many different body parts, different medications will be prescribed.

Some examples are medications that:.

**Vascular dilation:** Blood pressure medicines that do this may be able to treat Raynaud's syndrome.

Suppress the immune system: Immune-suppressive medications, such as those prescribed after organ transplants, may help slow the progression of some scleroderma symptoms, such as skin thickening or escalating lung damage.

**Reduce digestive symptoms:** Pills to lower stomach acid can help with heartburn relief. Bloating, diarrhea, and constipation may be lessened with the aid of antibiotics and drugs that facilitate the movement of food through the intestines.

**Prevent infections:** Cleaning and protection from the cold may help keep fingertip ulcers brought on by Raynaud's disease from getting infected. Immunizations against the flu and pneumonia on a regular basis can help protect lungs that have been harmed by scleroderma.

**Relieve pain:** If over-the-counter painkillers are insufficient, your doctor may recommend prescription painkillers.

## Therapies

Your strength and mobility can be improved, and you can maintain your independence with daily tasks with the aid of physical or occupational therapy. Hand therapy might help prevent contractures of the hands.

# Procedures, both medical and otherwise

For those whose severe symptoms have not improved with more conventional treatments, stem cell transplants may be an option. Organ transplants might be a possibility if the kidneys or lungs have suffered severe damage.

- A bone-marrow transplant.
- transplant of a kidney
- A lung transplant.

Although the cause of this particular reaction is unknown, the immune system is thought to be responsible.

Some people's scleroderma may also have a genetic component.

It is false to say that the disease is caused by the genetic component.

Instead, it is believed that it is set off when a person is exposed to specific toxic chemicals, like pesticides and solvents.

**Lifestyle and home remedies.**
You can take the following actions to help manage your scleroderma symptoms:.


• Keep on moving.

• Exercise promotes circulation, keeps your body flexible, and reduces stiffness.

With range-of-motion exercises, you can keep your skin and joints flexible. This is important at all times, but it is particularly important when the disease is first developing.

Use lotion and sunscreen frequently to take care of dry or stiff skin. Avoid hot baths and showers, strong soaps, and household chemicals because they can irritate and dry out your skin even more.

**No smoking:** Nicotine narrows blood vessels, which makes Raynaud's disease worse. Smoking can also cause permanent blood vessel narrowing, as well as create or exacerbate lung conditions.

To stop smoking, it can be difficult to ask your doctor for help.

**Treat heartburn as needed.**
Reduce your intake of the foods that give you heartburn or gas. Additionally, refrain from eating after midnight. To avoid experiencing esophageal reflux while you sleep, raise the head of your bed. Antacids may offer symptom relief.

Avoid coming into contact with the cold by always wearing warm mittens to protect your hands, even when reaching into a freezer. It's essential to keep your body's core temperature warm in order to lessen the effects of Raynaud's. When you're outside in the cold, dress in layers of warm clothing, keep your face and head covered, and wear warm boots.

# Scleroderma Treatment Naturally.

A rare, chronic autoimmune connective tissue disease called scleroderma causes the skin and connective tissues to tighten and harden. Scleroderma can be treated naturally by balancing the biochemistry of the gut and blood, calming the immune system, avoiding triggers, and reducing stress.

Everybody is affected, including Perth, Australia.

Scleroderma is derived from the Greek words for "hard skin" and "sclero.".

When the immune system attacks itself, a condition known as an autoimmune disorder, such as scleroderma, results. The immune system safeguards the body as it should by warding off external invaders like viruses and infections. As a result of the immune system mistakenly attacking the body's own tissues as foreign invaders in autoimmune disease, a variety of complications can result.

Scleroderma patients experience inflammation as a result of the immune system attack, which also causes the body to produce an excessive amount of collagen as if there were an injury that needs to be repaired. The extra collagen in the tissues can affect how well the body's organs work normally. Too much collagen can cause skin to become tight and hard, and occasionally internal organs as well. [2] It is unclear to scientists what triggers this autoimmune response. Both the environment and genetics might be significant.

69

There is a wide range of symptoms that scleroderma patients can experience, from very minor problems in some to very serious illnesses in others. Most patients suffer from the milder condition.

Scleroderma can seriously harm your kidneys, oesophagus, lungs, heart, and digestive system. It is not infectious, cancerous, or malignant, but it has the potential to be fatal. It may also lead to other health issues such as kidney failure, muscle disorders, cancer, heart failure, pulmonary fibrosis, high blood pressure in the lungs (pulmonary hypertension), problems absorbing nutrients from food, and kidney failure. Natural remedies can be used to treat scleroderma symptoms and prevent the immune system from overreacting, which aggravates the condition.

Developing the condition is possible if you:.

using bleomycin and other specific chemotherapy drugs.

being exposed to silica dust and organic solvents.


## Variations on scleroderma

There are two types of scleroderma: systemic and localized.

Only a person's skin may occasionally be affected by scleroderma.

This is known medically as localized scleroderma.

Some people with scleroderma may also experience damage to blood vessels, internal organs, and the digestive system.

This is referred to in medicine as systemic scleroderma.

## Just a localized form of scleroderma

Localized, usually mild scleroderma affects about 70% of people. It only impacts the skin, despite the fact that it can spread to the muscles, joints, and bones. Localized scleroderma rarely progresses to a systemic condition and hardly ever affects the internal organs.

One of two forms of localized scleroderma is possible:.

**Morphea:** This occurs when skin patches of various colors appear. These patches have various shapes, colors, and sizes and have a waxy appearance.

Linear scleroderma: This condition results in bands or streaks of thick, hard skin on the arms and legs. The term "en coup de sabre" is used when streaks appear on the head or neck. It was given that name because it resembles a saber or sword wound.

**Scleroderma systemica.**
Systemic scleroderma falls into two main classifications: diffuse and limited.

The signs and symptoms of systemic scleroderma include skin tightening and thickening that appears more quickly and in more skin areas than in limited scleroderma. In addition to the skin, muscles, joints, bones, blood vessels, heart, gastrointestinal tract, oesophagus, lungs, and kidneys, it also affects the connective tissue in many other parts of the body.

## Scleroderma diffuse

Many body parts are affected by this form.

It can harm many internal organs in addition to the skin, impairing breathing and digestion while also increasing the risk of kidney failure. Sometimes, systemic scleroderma can develop into a serious and even fatal condition.

If you have symptoms in your internal organs that start to harden, this is the most severe type. This form is present in about 30% of patients.

**Scleroderma with limited severity**

Limited scleroderma is sometimes referred to as "CREST," which is an acronym for five of the condition's most noticeable symptoms.

Calcinosis is a condition wherein calcium deposits under the skin of the fingers and other parts of the body cause small, white lumps to appear.

When exposed to cold temperatures or stress, body parts, such as the fingers and toes, become numb and cold (Raynaud phenomenon). This results from restricted blood flow after smaller arteries that supply blood to the skin start to narrow.

**Esophageal dysfunction:** When the skin in the esophagus hardens, it reduces the function of the muscles and makes swallowing more challenging.

**Sclerodactyly:** When a buildup of fibrous tissue causes the skin to tighten so much that you can no longer curl your fingers and you lose mobility.

**Telangiectasia:** The development of threadlike red lines on the skin as a result of dilated blood vessels close to the skin's surface.

Renal issues are not present in people with limited scleroderma.

Fingers, hands, forearms, feet, and legs are the only body parts where the skin is thickening. Generally speaking, only the oesophagus is involved in digestion. Pulmonary hypertension, which can manifest in 20% to 30% of cases, is one of the more serious late complications.

## Scleroderma signs and symptoms and natural treatments for the condition

Depending on the type of scleroderma you have and the organs it has affected, there are different signs and symptoms. These signs may appear as:

In the early stages of the condition, systemic scleroderma may only impact the skin. Around your mouth, nose, fingers, and other bony areas, you might notice that your skin is getting thicker and developing shiny spots.

You might experience restricted movement in the affected areas as the condition worsens.

Other signs include:

- loss of hair
- Under the skin, there may be calcium deposits or white lumps
- Under the skin's surface, there are little, dilated blood vessels
- joint discomfort
- breathing difficulty
- an unproductive cough
- diarrhea
- constipation
- a problem swallowing
- Reflux of the esophagus.
- stomach bloating following a meal

The blood vessels in your fingers and toes may spasm due to the Raynaud's phenomenon. Then, when you are exposed to extreme cold or emotional stress, your extremities may turn white and blue.

## Scleroderma Treatment through Natural Means

There are a number of things you can do to manage your scleroderma; natural treatments for scleroderma include:

Avoid exposure to cold temperatures, dress warmly, and avoid smoking as these all worsen the Raynaud's phenomenon.

Include regular, light exercise in your daily routine to maintain the mobility of your joints, enhance blood circulation, build up your muscles, and enhance your general health.

It will be easier for you to handle the demands and difficulties of the condition if you can control your stress.

- Take a lot of naps.
- Obtain plenty of liquids.
- Put on lotions made of shea butter or raw coconut oil.
- To maintain flexible skin and joints, practice yoga and gentle stretches.
- Eat a balanced diet to help maintain your weight, give you more energy, and improve your overall wellbeing.
- To enable optimum immune function, heal your gut and balance your microbiome. To help keep your digestive system healthy, take a

probiotic supplement containing Lactobacillus acidophilus or bifidobacterium.

- Eliminate gluten-containing grains and legumes from your diet because they cause inflammation, which results in leaky gut. Removing dairy products can also help some people with their symptoms, according to some. consuming a diet that is AIP.

- Use the potent antioxidant glutathione to promote detoxification. Scleroderma incidence and toxic chemicals have been linked, according to research.

- Ensure adequate vitamin D intake. In a study of 51 patients conducted in 2016, researchers found that systemic sclerosis frequently has low vitamin

D levels. The authors came to the conclusion that having low vitamin levels may be associated with a more severe disease that involves multiple visceral organs, especially the heart and lungs.

- Make sure you're getting enough vitamin E

Every day, consume omega-3 fatty acids, such as fish oil. A few studies indicate that omega-3 fatty acids may lessen Raynaud's phenomenon symptoms and help people better withstand cold temperatures. They also help to improve blood flow. Halibut and salmon are two excellent sources of cold-water fish.

- Circulation can be enhanced by physical therapy and massage.

- Take bromelain, which can help decrease inflammation and pain.

- Turmeric can be taken to ease pain and reduce inflammation.

- Take gotu kola to promote circulation and healthy blood vessels. Scleroderma symptoms may be lessened by some gotu kola purified extracts.

## Scleroderma

A group of illnesses known as scleroderma make skin hard and constrictive, as well as occasionally internal organs. Actually, the word "scleroderma" means "hard skin.". The protein collagen, which makes up connective tissues, is overproduced by the body, which causes it to occur

The hands and face are typically the only body parts where localized scleroderma manifests. Scleroderma that affects the connective tissue in many areas of your body, including your internal organs, is called systemic scleroderma.

Scleroderma is regarded as an autoimmune condition, which means that the body's own tissues are mistakenly attacked by the immune system. 300,000 Americans are estimated to suffer from scleroderma, according to the Scleroderma Foundation. In women than in men, it occurs more frequently.

## Symptoms and indications

Scleroderma symptoms could include the following:

## Restricted scleroderma

**Morphea scleroderma**: Oval, thick patches of skin that are white in the center and purple around the edges. In addition to the arms and legs, they can also be found on the chest, back, and stomach.

Streaks of hardened skin that appear on the arms, legs, or forehead are known as linear scleroderma.

## Scleroderma systemica

Skin on the fingers, hands, arms, legs, face, neck, and trunk hardens due to diffuse cutaneous systemic sclerosis. Both sides of the body are typically affected by this type of scleroderma, so if your left arm is bothering you, your right arm probably does too. It may also have an impact on the heart, lungs, kidneys, and esophagus, among other internal organs.

Systemic sclerosis with limited cutaneous involvement: Affects the skin on the face, neck, lower arms, and fingers. CREST syndrome is a common symptom in people with this type of scleroderma. The acronym CREST stands for:

- Calcium deposits under the skin that cause pain are called calcinosis.
- Sensitivity to cold in the hands and feet, or Raynaud's phenomenon.
- difficulties swallowing due to internal scarring, or esophageal dysfunction.
- Sclerodactyly, a tightening of the skin on the fingers or toes.

- Blood vessels on the face, lips, forearms, hands, and palms swell, a condition known as telangiectasia.
- Internal organs are affected by sine scleroderma, but not the skin.
- headaches as well as seizures.

## Causes

The immune system mistakenly attacking the body's own tissues is thought by doctors to be the cause of scleroderma. The body produces too much collagen as a result of the immune system attack, which also causes inflammation. Skin that has too much collagen becomes tight and hard, and occasionally so do internal organs. What sets off this autoimmune response is unknown to researchers. Environment and genetics may both be important.

Scleroderma risk may be raised by the following factors:

## Diagnosis

Scleroderma is not always simple to diagnose. Rheumatologists (who specialize in treating arthritis) and dermatologists (who specialize in treating skin conditions) may both be needed. The doctor will perform a physical examination and feel your skin to look for areas of hardening and thickening. The physician may also apply pressure to the tendons and joints that are hurt:

- blood tests to check for higher immune system-produced antibody levels.
- Skin biopsy is used to diagnose skin issues.

- To evaluate lung damage, have a chest X-ray or a pulmonary function test.

- To determine if the muscles and internal organs have been harmed, an MRI or CT scan may be used.

Many of the initial symptoms of scleroderma resemble those of other connective-tissue disorders, including lupus, polymyositis, and rheumatoid arthritis. Mixed connective-tissue disease is the name given when a person has more than one of these conditions.

## Care for the future.

Although there is no known way to prevent scleroderma, there are precautions you can take to keep from getting infections if you already have the condition. Your physician might suggest that.

## Pneumococcal vaccine for pneumonia

- flu shot every year.

## Treatment

Scleroderma does not have a treatment.

Drugs can treat symptoms and shield against complications. Making lifestyle and dietary adjustments can make living with the disease easier.

## Lifestyle.

It might be possible to improve quality of life by taking these straightforward steps:

- To lessen gas or heartburn, eat small, frequent meals

- Maintaining flexibility in the joints and skin through exercise

- DON'T SMOKE, as tobacco worsens scleroderma

- Avoid stress and cold exposure because they can impair circulation

- To lessen discomfort, stiffness, and swelling, apply calming skin creams.

## Medication

Doctors frequently use steroid creams or moisturizers to treat localized scleroderma. If localized scleroderma affects a large area of the body, such as the entire arm or leg, oral medications, such as minocycline

(Minocin or Dynacin), may also be used to prevent it from getting worse.

Medication that enhances circulation, lowers heartburn, protects kidney function, and regulates high blood pressure may be used to treat systemic scleroderma. The following are some drugs that a doctor might suggest for scleroderma.

**Nonsteroidal anti-inflammatory drugs (NSAIDs):** NSAIDs are medications that reduce pain and inflammation in the joints.

Drugs that increase circulation can lower the signs and symptoms of scleroderma and lower blood pressure. They are as follows:

- CCBs (calcium channel blockers)
- Anti-angiotensin II receptor drugs
- inhibitors of the angiotensin-converting enzyme (ACE)
- Alpha obstructors
- Aspirin

Disease-modifying antirheumatic medications (DMARDs): DMARDs slow the disease's progression.

They are as follows:

- Plaquenil (hydroxychloroquinine).
- (Rheumatrex) methotrexate.

Azulfidine, also known as sulfasalazine.

**Immunosuppressants:** Reduce the immune system's overactivity.

Kidney damage and an increased risk of infection are just two of the serious side effects that these medications may cause. They are as follows:

- Imuran, or azathioprine.
- Cytoxan (Cyclophosphamide).
- Closporin (Neoral).

**Antacids:** To lessen heartburn when the esophagus is injured.

## Surgery and additional procedures

Doctors may advise the following procedures when scleroderma symptoms are very severe:

- abdominal or intestinal wall repair surgery.
- An amputation of a finger or toe that is severely ill and infected.

- Rare cases may involve lung, heart, or kidney transplants.

- food supplements and nutrition.

Scleroderma sufferers might not consume enough vitamins and minerals, especially if their digestive systems are damaged. You might be advised to take a supplement by your doctor. Always be honest with your doctor about any herbs and supplements you use or are thinking about using.

Especially if you have a chronic illness, these general nutritional advices are beneficial for your overall health.

- Consume foods high in antioxidants, such as bell peppers and squash, as well as fruits and vegetables (such as blueberries, cherries, and tomatoes).

- Avoid refined foods, especially sugar and white breads, pastas, and pasta sauces.

- Lean meats, cold-water fish, tofu (soy, if no allergies), or beans should be consumed more often than red meat.

- Use wholesome oils like olive or vegetable.

- Reduce or eliminate trans fatty acids, which are present in processed foods and commercially baked goods like cookies, crackers, cakes, French fries, onion rings, and donuts

- Don't use alcohol, tobacco, or caffeine

- Every day, chug six to eight glasses of filtered water

- 5 days a week, spend at least 30 minutes a day working out

The antioxidant vitamins A, C, and E, the B-complex vitamins, and trace minerals like magnesium, calcium, zinc, and selenium may be included in a daily multivitamin that your doctor suggests taking.

Some of the symptoms may be lessened with the aid of these supplements:

1 to 2 capsules or 1 to 3 tablespoons of omega-3 fatty acids, such as fish oil. of oil, 1–3 times per day. A few studies indicate that omega-3 fatty acids may lessen Raynaud's phenomenon symptoms and help people better tolerate cold temperatures in addition to helping blood flow.

Salmon and halibut are excellent sources of cold-water fish.

You run a higher risk of bleeding if you take omega-3 supplements.

Consult your doctor before taking omega-3 supplements if you take blood thinners like aspirin, clopidogrel, or warfarin (Coumadin).


**Bromelain**
Bromelain helps lessen pain and inflammation even though it is not a treatment for scleroderma.

It frequently goes together with turmeric.

A variety of medications and bromelain may interact.

Ask your doctor before taking bromelain if you take blood thinners like warfarin (Coumadin), clopidogrel (Plavix), or aspirin because it may increase your risk of bleeding.

A probiotic supplement with 5 to 10 billion CFUs (colony forming units) per day, preferably one with Lactobacillus acidophilus or Bifidobacterium. These "friendly" bacteria assist in maintaining digestive health. According to one study, probiotics helped people with scleroderma who experienced digestive system-related bloating feel less uncomfortable. Before taking probiotics, make sure to consult your doctor because some studies suggest they may be problematic for people with autoimmune diseases or compromised immune systems.

## Herbs

Systems in the body may be strengthened and toned by herbs.

You should consult with your doctor before beginning therapy, as with any therapy.

The use of herbs to treat scleroderma has not been extensively studied.

Prior to taking any supplements or herbs, consult your doctor.

## The longa species of turmeric

Turmeric reduces inflammation, according to lab studies.

Although more research is required to determine whether it is effective for scleroderma, it may also help with pain management.

Bromelain is frequently added to it.

The risk of bleeding may be increased by turmeric.

Consult your doctor before taking turmeric if you take blood thinners like aspirin, clopidogrel, or warfarin (Coumadin).

For the health and circulation of the blood vessels, use gotu kola (Centella asiatica). The symptoms of scleroderma appear to be lessened by some gotu kola purified extracts. More investigation is required. Gotu kola may have an effect on the liver and interact with sedative medications. Before consuming gotu kola, consult your doctor.

## Acupuncture

A few studies indicate that acupuncture may enhance blood flow to the hands and fingers, aid in the recovery of fingertip ulcers, and possibly lessen the development of fibrous tissue. It might also reduce pain.

## Physiotherapy and massage

Massage may aid in improving circulation, according to research.

If massage helps people with scleroderma, more study is required.

## Body-Mind Medicine

Despite conflicting research, biofeedback may help some scleroderma patients better regulate the temperature in their hands and feet. Counseling, meditation, and other mind-body practices like the emotional freedom technique (EFT) may also be beneficial.

# VARIOUS OTHER FACTORS

## Complications and prognosis

For the first few years in some people, symptoms appear quickly and worsen over time. But for the majority of patients, the illness worsens gradually over time.

The outlook is better for those with only skin symptoms. Scleroderma that is widespread (systemic) can cause:

- Muscle problems.
- Cancer.
- failure of the heart.
- Pulmonary fibrosis is the term for lung scarring

- Pulmonary hypertension: high blood pressure in the lungs
- kidney malfunction
- issues with food's nutritional absorption

Skin and other body parts become inflamed as a result of the connective tissue and rheumatic autoimmune disease known as scleroderma. Scleroderma develops when an immune response misleads tissues into believing they are injured, triggering inflammation and an overproduction of collagen in the body. Patches of tight, hard skin develop as a result of excessive collagen in your skin and other tissues. Numerous body systems are affected by scleroderma. You can better understand how the disease impacts each of those systems by using the definitions that follow.

A connective tissue disease is one that affects tissues like the skin, tendons, and cartilage. Other tissues and organs are supported, shielded, and given structure by connective tissue.

When the immune system, which normally aids in protecting the body from infection and disease, attacks its own tissues, autoimmune diseases are the result.

A group of diseases collectively referred to as rheumatic diseases are characterized by inflammation or pain in the muscles, joints, or fibrous tissue.

Scleroderma comes in two main types:

Scleroderma that is localized only affects the skin and the tissues underneath the skin.

Systemic sclerosis, also known as systemic scleroderma, has an impact on a variety of bodily systems. Scleroderma of this severity can harm your blood vessels and internal organs, including the heart, lungs, and kidneys.

## Scleroderma does not have a treatment

Relieving symptoms and halting the spread of the disease are the objectives of treatment. The importance of early diagnosis and ongoing monitoring cannot be overstated.

## What occurs with scleroderma?

Scleroderma has no known cause. However, scientists believe that the immune system overreacts, resulting in inflammation and damage to the blood vessel lining cells. This prompts the production of excessive amounts of collagen and other proteins by connective tissue cells, especially a cell type known as fibroblasts. The abnormally long-lived fibroblasts result in a buildup of collagen in the skin and other organs, which causes the scleroderma symptoms and signs to manifest.

## Who is prone to scleroderma?
Scleroderma can affect anyone, but some populations are more likely to get it than others.

You may be at risk if the following things happen.

## Sex

Women experience scleroderma more frequently than men do.

**Age:** The illness typically strikes between the ages of 30 and 50, striking adults more frequently than children.

## Race

All racial and ethnic groups are susceptible to scleroderma, but African Americans are more likely to be severely affected by the condition. For example:

African Americans are more likely to contract the illness than are European Americans.

Comparatively speaking to other groups, African Americans who have scleroderma experience the disease's onset earlier.

Compared to other groups, African Americans are more likely to have lung disease and skin involvement.

## Various Scleroderma types

Localized scleroderma typically manifests in one or both of these patterns, affecting the skin and underlying tissues.

Morphea, or scleroderma patches that may measure half an inch or more in diameter.

Scleroderma that thickens in a straight line. This typically runs down a leg or arm, but it can also occur on the forehead and face.

Your skin, tissues, blood vessels, and major organs are all impacted by systemic scleroderma, also known as systemic sclerosis. Systemic scleroderma is typically divided into two categories by doctors:.

Skin on your fingers, hands, face, lower arms, and legs below the knees is affected by limited cutaneous scleroderma, which develops gradually.

When it first begins, diffuse cutaneous scleroderma only affects the fingers and toes.

However, as it progresses, it affects the upper arms, trunk, and thighs in addition to the elbows and knees.

Internal organ damage is more common with this type.

## Scleroderma signs and symptoms

Depending on the type of scleroderma you have, your specific symptoms will vary from person to person.

- Patches of thick, hard skin typically appear in one of two patterns with localized scleroderma.
- Skin patches that have morphea thicken into firm, oval-shaped areas.
- These spots could have a waxy, yellow appearance with a reddish or bruise-like edge.
- The patches could stay in one spot or spread to other skin types

- Over time, the disease usually becomes dormant, but you might still have skin patches that are darker than usual
- Additionally, some individuals experience fatigue

Your arm, leg, and, in rare cases, your forehead develop thickened or discolored lines due to linear scleroderma.

Systemic sclerosis, also known as systemic scleroderma, can develop suddenly or gradually and can affect your internal organs in addition to your skin.

Frustration is a common symptom of this kind of scleroderma.

Scleroderma that only affects the skin on your fingers, hands, face, lower arms, and legs below the knees typically develops gradually. Additionally, it may result in issues with your esophagus and blood vessels. Although internal organs are affected by the limited form, it generally isn't as severe as the diffuse form. The symptoms known as CREST, which stands for the following symptoms, are frequently present in people with limited cutaneous scleroderma.

Calcinosis, which can be seen on an x-ray, is the formation of calcium deposits in the connective tissues.

In Raynaud's phenomenon, the small blood vessels in the hands or feet constrict in response to cold or stress, changing the color of the fingers and toes to white, blue, and/or red.

Esophageal dysfunction, also known as impaired esophageal function, is brought on when the smooth muscles in the esophagus stop moving normally.

The esophagus is the tube that connects the throat and the stomach.

The excessive collagen deposits within the skin layers cause sclerodactyly, which is the thick, tight skin on the fingers.

Small red spots appear on the hands and face as a result of the condition telangiectasia, which is brought on by the swelling of tiny blood vessels.

Skin thickening on your fingers or toes is typically the first symptom of diffuse cutaneous scleroderma, which develops suddenly. Over your elbows and/or knees, the thickening of the skin then spreads to the rest of your body. This kind may harm your internal organs, including:

- any location along your digestive tract
- your respiratory system
- kidneys in you
- a part of you

CREST features can also be present in diffuse scleroderma patients, despite the term's historical association with the limited form of the disease.

## Scleroderma causes

Scleroderma's exact cause is unknown, but researchers believe that a number of factors may be involved in the development of the condition:

## Genetic make-up

Scleroderma can be hereditarily predisposed in some individuals, and the type of scleroderma they have can also be influenced by genetics. The illness cannot be inherited, and unlike some genetic illnesses, it is not passed from parent to child. However, compared to the general population, first-degree relatives of scleroderma patients have a higher risk of contracting the disease.

## Environment

Scleroderma may be brought on by exposure to certain environmental factors like viruses or chemicals, according to researchers.

Immune system modifications. Your body's abnormal immune or inflammatory activity sets off cellular alterations that result in an excessive amount of collagen being produced.

## Hormones

The majority of scleroderma types affect women more frequently than they do men. According to researchers, the disease may be influenced by hormonal variations between men and women.

## What scleroderma symptoms are present?

There are numerous signs and symptoms of scleroderma.

You can see a few of the effects it can have on your skin in the following pictures.

117

- Skin that is getting harder or tighter.

- Scleroderma is named for this characteristic. Some individuals get one or two patches of thick, hard skin. Others have body-wide patches. The thick, hard skin can make one feel firmly planted. The most prevalent form of scleroderma, morphea (more-fee-uh), causes patches that are not always painful. The brittle skin might soften over time.

- arm patches with scleroderma.

- less sweating and hair loss.

- It's common to notice shiny, discolored, and thinning hair where your skin has hardened. The skin's tendency to stop sweating is another sign of its hardening.

- Foot and lower leg have linear morphea.

- Itches and dry skin.

- Extremely dry skin, which itches, is a side effect of scleroderma. The skin may break down as a result of the extreme dryness, and sores may develop.

- Man scratching his forearm.

- Skin tone varies

- Patches of skin that have hardened can be lighter or darker than your actual skin tone. When scleroderma is active and growing, some people experience violet-colored skin. This patient has hard-to-touch darker and lighter (white) areas.

- On the woman's lower back, there are scleroderma patches of aged skin.

- The skin has a salt-and-pepper appearance.

The upper back, chest, or scalp (along the hairline) are the typical sites for this to appear. Although not always, the skin may feel stiff or constrictive. You should see a doctor if your skin has a salt-and-pepper appearance. This might indicate that you have an internal organ-affecting form of scleroderma. Your prognosis (what is likely to happen) will be better if you receive treatment and a diagnosis quickly.

A salt-and-pepper appearance to the skin can be brought on by scleroderma.

joints that are difficult to move and are stiff.

When the skin over a joint becomes tight, thick, or hard (i.e. e. It may be challenging to move that joint (for example, the jaw, wrist, or finger) due to the tightness. The patient in this image has skin that is too tight for her to fully open her hands. You can keep your entire range of motion with the aid of physical therapy. Without it, you might not be able to fully straighten or bend your finger, wrist, elbow, or other part of your body.

Due to diffuse cutaneous scleroderma, the woman is unable to straighten her fingers.

## Weakening and shortening of muscles

Sometimes the muscle is affected by the hardening and tightening. The muscle may become shorter and weaker as a result. It's possible that you can't stretch the muscle.

It's important to let your doctor know if you experience muscle wasting so that the underlying problem can be identified and treated.

## Muscles that hurt

the destruction of skin-deep tissue.

A form of scleroderma known as Parry-Romberg syndrome (PRS) affects this girl, and it can result in bone, cartilage, and muscle loss. As seen here, PRS typically only affects one side of the face. It can also impact the trunk, a leg, or an arm. A very uncommon condition, PRS. Tissue loss beneath the skin is a side effect of other types of scleroderma.

- muscle and tissue loss due to scleroderma
- Bone may not develop as it ought to
- Certain types of scleroderma, like linear scleroderma and en coup de sabre, can prevent a child's bones from growing
- A leg might not grow as it ought to
- Scleroderma that affects the head may cause facial deformity
- These anomalies are uncommon
- Scleroderma-related bone deformity
- On the fingers, there are sores and scars with pits

Skin sores are frequently present in individuals who suffer from a form of scleroderma that also impacts the internal organs. The skin that has been stretched tightly tends to develop these sores. On the fingers, sores are particularly typical. On their fingertips and the sides of their fingers, some people get pitted scars that are the size of a pinhead.

Treprostinil was tested in a pilot study on systemic sclerosis patients to see if it could treat and prevent digital ulcers.

Scleroderma patient's fingers have sores and pitted scars.

deposits of calcium under the skin.

This condition, known as calcinosis (KAL-sin-OH-sis), develops in the connective tissue under the skin. You might feel one or more painful, hard lumps under your skin. A calcium deposit that penetrates the skin can be extremely painful and cause a white or yellow chalky substance to appear. Open sores may become painful and infected.

Scleroderma-related finger sores and calcium buildup.

## Present blood vessels

Small blood vessels close to the skin's surface swell, causing this to happen. Tiny red spots, typically on the hands and face, could be seen. Although it is not painful, many people do not like how these appear. There is care available.

Scleroderma-induced visible blood vessels on the palm of the hand.

extraordinary sensitivity to stress, the cold, or both.

This is frequently a sign of internal organ damage from scleroderma.

This symptom is referred to in medicine as Raynaud's phenomenon. When it's cold outside or you're under stress, it makes some parts of your body—typically the fingers, toes, ears, or tip of your nose—feel cold and turn numb. You might experience white and then blue skin. The affected areas frequently turn red as the blood flow resumes normal.

## Scleroderma is not always a part of Raynaud's disease

However, scleroderma patients may experience issues due to the restricted blood flow. The skin on the fingers may become sore or pitted as a result of Raynaud's disease.

Scleroderma is a condition where fibrous tissue accumulates in the skin and other parts of the body. Additionally, it harms the cells that line the walls of small arteries. As a result of the inadequate blood supply, tissue damage results.

## Various Names

Progressive systemic sclerosis, Systemic sclerosis, Limited scleroderma, CREST syndrome, Localized scleroderma, Linear morphea, Raynaud's phenomenon - scleroderma.

## Causes

An example of an autoimmune disorder is scleroderma. This condition occurs when the immune system unintentionally targets and harms healthy body tissue.

## Scleroderma doesn't have a known cause

The disease's symptoms are brought on by an accumulation of a substance called collagen in the skin and other organs.

People between the ages of 30 and 50 are most frequently affected by the disease. Scleroderma affects more women than men. Some people with scleroderma have a history of exposure to silica dust and polyvinyl chloride, but most do not.

Systemic lupus erythematosus, polymyositis, and widespread scleroderma are autoimmune conditions that can co-occur. Undifferentiated connective tissue disease or overlap syndrome are the terms used to describe these conditions.

## Symptoms

Scleroderma can affect the whole body or just the skin in some cases.

Localized scleroderma, also known as morphea, typically only affects the skin on the chest, abdomen, or limbs and rarely the hands or the face. Morphea develops gradually and rarely spreads throughout the body or leads to serious issues like damage to internal organs.

Sclerosis, also known as systemic scleroderma, can affect the heart, lungs, kidneys, and large regions of skin. Limited disease (CREST syndrome) and diffuse disease are the two main types.

# CREST condition

Scleroderma skin symptoms could include:

- the Raynaud phenomenon, whereby fingers or toes turn blue or white in response to cold temperatures.

- Skin on the fingers, hands, forearm, and face feels tight and rigid.

- loss of hair.

- Skin that is lighter or darker than usual.

- Under the skin, there are tiny, white calcium crystals that occasionally ooze a toothpaste-like substance

- toes or fingernails with sores (ulcers)

- Face skin that's constricted and mask-like

- Telangiectasias are tiny, widened blood vessels that are visible beneath the skin on the face or at the base of fingernails

Symptoms involving bones and muscles could be:

- Motion is lost as a result of joint stiffness, pain, and swelling. Due to fibrosis around tissue and tendons, the hands are frequently involved.
- feet that are numb and hurt

Scarring in the lungs can cause breathing issues, which can include the following.

- coughing up dry.
- breathing difficulty
- Wheezing
- risk of lung cancer increasing

among the issues with the digestive system are:

- swallowing issues

- heartburn or esophageal reflux

- post-meal bloating

- Constipation

## Diarrhea

- issues with stool control.

- Some potential heart issues are:.

- irregular heartbeat.

- The heart's surrounding fluid.

- Heart function is reduced due to fibrosis in the heart muscle.

- among other things, kidney and genitourinary issues could be.

- kidney failure beginning to develop.

- erection problems in men

- Vaginal dryness in females

## Testing and Exams

The doctor will perform a thorough physical examination. The examination could reveal:

- the face, fingers, or other areas with tight, thick skin
- In order to check for abnormalities of the small blood vessels, the skin at the base of the fingernails can be viewed through a lit magnifying glass.
- There will be a check for anomalies in the abdomen, heart, and lungs
- Your blood pressure will be measured. Small blood vessels in the kidneys may narrow as a result of scleroderma. High blood pressure and decreased kidney function are

both consequences of kidney problems

**Tests using blood and urine could include:**

**ANA panel:** a list of antinuclear antibodies.

- Antibody testing for scleroderma.
- ESR stands for heart rate.
- Factor rheumatoid
- total count of the blood
- metabolic panel with creatinine included
- tests of the heart's muscles
- Urinalysis

Additional tests might consist of:.

- imaging of the chest.

- lungs' CT scan
- (ECG) Electrocardiogram
- Echocardiogram

## Examinations to determine the health of your digestive system and lungs.

A skin biopsy

## Treatment

Scleroderma doesn't have a specific treatment. The severity of disease in the skin, lungs, kidneys, heart, and gastrointestinal tract will be evaluated by your healthcare provider.

Individuals with widespread skin disease (as opposed to localized skin involvement) may be more susceptible to internal organ and progressive diseases. Diffuse cutaneous systemic sclerosis (dcSSc) is the official name for this variation of the illness. This group of patients typically receives body-wide (systemic) treatments.

To manage your symptoms and avoid complications, you will be given medications and other treatments.

The following medications are used to treat progressive scleroderma.

- Prednisone is an example of a corticosteroid. However, doses above 10 mg per day are not advised because higher doses may result in kidney disease and high blood pressure.

- Immune system-suppressing medications like methotrexate, cyclophosphamide, cyclosporine, and mycophenolate.

- Treatment of arthritis with hydroxychloroquine.

- HSCT using autologous hematopoietic stem cells may be an option for some people with scleroderma that is rapidly progressing. In specialized facilities, this kind of treatment must be administered

The following additional treatments are possible for particular symptoms:

- Raynaud's phenomenon treatments

- medications for heartburn or swallowing issues, such as omeprazole

- For high blood pressure or kidney issues, blood pressure medications are available, such as ACE inhibitors

- Skin thickening can be treated with light therapy

- Bosentan and sildenafil are two examples of drugs that help the lungs function better

## Treatment options for scleroderma

Understanding your disease subtype, stage, and involved organs is crucial in figuring out the best course of treatment for Scleroderma because no two cases are exactly alike. The four primary aspects of the disease—inflammation, autoimmunity, vascular disease, and tissue fibrosis—are the focus of the current treatments, which include pharmaceuticals. The best treatments for you will be determined by your doctor and you; however, the following are some frequent options:.

## MEDICINES THAT ARE ANTI-INFLAMMATORY

Many drugs are thought to either directly or indirectly reduce inflammation. There are two main types of inflammation in scleroderma that are connected to the illness process. The first is a more common type that can result in arthritis (joint inflammation), myositis (muscle inflammation), or serositis (inflammation of the heart's or lung's lining, respectively).

139

NSAIDs (e.g., aspirin) are effective at treating this kind of inflammation.

either ibuprofen or corticosteroids (e. g. prednisone). The particular circumstance determines how long therapy will last and how much medication to take. Some patients will require ongoing care, while others will recover after only a brief course of therapy.

The skin and other tissues that have been harmed by the scleroderma process are the subject of the other type of inflammation. NSAIDs and corticosteroids do not seem to help this stage of the disease, though the precise function of corticosteroids is not well understood. The use of these medications carries some risks, such as renal toxicity, fluid retention, and gastrointestinal disease. An increased risk of renal crisis in scleroderma is also linked to corticosteroid use. The use of NSAIDs and corticosteroids is therefore advised to be restricted to inflammatory conditions that exhibit responsiveness.


**Therapeutical Immunosuppression**
Immunosuppressive therapy is the most widely used method of managing the inflammatory stage of scleroderma. The theory goes that the inflammation is brought on by an autoimmune process, and that tissue damage and fibrosis follow as a consequence. According to this theory, fibrosis is an "innocent bystander" that is fueled by cytokines, which are chemical messengers created by the immune system. Despite the fact that many different

medications are in use, few well-designed studies have been carried out.

These immunosuppressive medications include cyclosporine, methotrexate, antithymocyte globulin, mycophenolate mofetil, and cyclophosphamide. According to a recent study, methotrexate did not significantly differ from placebo (no treatment) in the skin score, which is a gauge of skin thickening. Because of reports of renal toxicity, cyclosporine is not fully studied. Mycophenolate mofetil or cyclophosphamide with or without antithymocyte globulin are the most effective medications. Sadly, there isn't any research that was placebo-controlled (i.e., half the patients receive the medication, and half receive a sugar pill) to pinpoint exactly how they should be used to treat scleroderma, but when given during the disease's active inflammatory phase, they seem to be effective.

The use of aggressive immunosuppressive therapy, whether with autologous bone marrow transplantation or very high doses of cyclophosphamide, is a significant area of current research. Due to the potential risks associated with these aggressive immunosuppressive therapies, they should only be used in the most severe forms of scleroderma and given in accordance with a research protocol.

## Vascular Disease Drug Therapy

Small and medium arteries are both affected by the widespread vascular disease associated with scleroderma. Clinically, it appears as Raynaud's phenomenon in the skin, and there is proof that other tissues experience recurrent episodes of ischemia (low oxygen state). Low blood flow into the skin and tissues is thought to activate fibroblasts and encourage tissue fibrosis in addition to damaging tissue through a lack of nutrition and oxygen. As a result, controlling vascular disease is now thought to be essential for both preventing organ damage and the disease's overall progression. Vasospasm (spasm of blood vessels), proliferative vasculopathy (thickening of blood vessels), and thrombosis (blood clots) or structural occlusion of the vessel lumen (blockage of blood vessels) are the three main manifestations of vascular disease that may require treatment.

Drugs that dilate blood vessels are the most effective way to treat vasospasm. Calcium channel blockers, such as esomeprazole, continue to be the most popular and effective vasodilator therapy.

Studies show that the use of calcium channel blockers can lessen the frequency of digital ulcers and attacks of Raynaud's phenomenon. We now understand that every organ's microcirculation has a special system for managing its own blood supply. The sympathetic nervous system controls the flow of blood to the skin, while locally produced hormones like renin control the flow of blood to the kidneys and endothelin, prostaglandins, and nitric oxide control the flow of blood to the lungs.

Each affected organ can be treated with a very specific agent to reduce the effects of the scleroderma vascular disease. For instance, it has been reported that calcium channel blockers improve blood flow to the skin and heart; angiotensin converting enzyme inhibitors (ACE) inhibitors reverse the vasospasm of the scleroderma renal crisis; and bosentan (a new endothelin-1 receptor inhibitor) or epoprostenol (prostacyclin) enhance blood flow to the lungs.

There are a number of vasoactive medications on the market that are used to treat vascular disease, but none of them are known to reverse intimal proliferation, which is a feature of the vascular disease associated with scleroderma and involves the thickening of the blood vessel's inner layer. The potential exists to alter the course of the disease with vasospasm-reversing medications, such as prostacyclin, bosentan, calcium channel blockers, and nitric oxide. There is proof that these vasodilators could also have an impact on tissue fibrosis directly. For instance, the fact that bosentan blocks endothelin-1, a blood vessel-produced molecule that can also directly stimulate tissue fibroblasts to produce collagen, may be advantageous.

Untreated scleroderma vascular disease ultimately results in thrombus formation or advanced intimal fibrosis, which obstructs the vessels. Aspirin at a low dose as anti-platelet therapy is therefore advised. There are no reliable studies to determine the value of antiplatelet or anticoagulation therapy. Anticoagulation (the use of blood-thinning medications) is frequently used for a brief period in an acute digital ischemic crisis (the sudden onset of threatened loss of a digit).

The connective tissues become tighter and harder as a result of the skin condition scleroderma. Another name for it is chronic progressive disease. Scleroderma primarily comes in two forms: systemic and localized. Scleroderma can affect your skin locally, but it can also affect your blood vessels and internal organs, such as your heart and lungs, systemically. Thickened skin, cold toes or fingers that turn blue, white, or red, sores or ulcers on the fingertips, muscle weakness, swollen joints, pain in the joints, dry eyes, dry mouth, shortness of breath, heartburn, diarrhea, swelling, and weight loss are some of the signs and symptoms of Scleroderma that are frequently experienced by patients. In allopathic medicine, patients are given anti-inflammatory medications like aspirin, ibuprofen, and steroids for scleroderma patients, which is not the ideal treatment. Therefore, a patient should adhere to some of the home remedies that will manage this condition in order to get relief from its symptoms. Here are some natural treatments that can be used to treat this illness at its source:

## 1. Turmeric

An old-fashioned herb known for its anti-inflammatory, analgesic, and immune-modulating properties is turmeric. These herb's properties lessen joint pain, inflammation, and stiffness.

## How to apply

Pour a glass of hot cow's milk over a teaspoonful of pure turmeric powder. Take this milk once or twice each day.

Additionally, you can make pure turmeric into a powder and keep it in a container. A teaspoonful of this powder can be mixed with a glass of water or used in cooking.

## 2. Garlic

Heartburn, muscle weakness, swollen joints, and inflammation are all conditions that garlic treats. This herb is conveniently accessible at home. So use this herb naturally to treat your scleroderma symptoms.

## What to do

As soon as you wake up in the morning, chew one to two cloves of roasted garlic.

You can also make a paste of garlic herb and apply it to the skin's affected area. Leave this on the skin's affected area for 30 minutes, then rinse it off once a day with regular water.

## 3. Ginger

In patients with scleroderma, the herb ginger reduces pain brought on by prostaglandins. This herb exhibits strong anti-inflammatory and antioxidant properties.

**What to do**

Grate some fresh ginger and add two cups of water. This should be heated to the last cup. Drink this herbal tea once or twice a day after straining the mixture.

A fresh ginger juice can also be taken and taken once or twice daily.

## 4. Onion

The herb onion reduces scleroderma-related inflammation, stiffness, heartburn, muscle weakness, joint pain, and other symptoms. Cepaene and thiosulfinates, two compounds abundant in onions that have anti-inflammatory properties. Scleroderma patients who use these properties experience less swelling and inflammation.

## What to do

Apply onion extract to the scleroderma area that is affected for 30 minutes. Then, wash this off with some regular water.

This herb can be added to food as a cooking ingredient.

## 5. Gotukola

The herb gotukola is effective at easing the signs and symptoms experienced by people with scleroderma.

It keeps the body's blood vessels healthy and improves circulation generally.

## How to apply

Take some fresh gotukola leaves and boil them in two cups of water for the remaining half cup. Take a few sips of this herbal tea every day after straining the mixture.

The market offers capsules containing the standardized extract of the herb gotu kola.

Each day, take one capsule with a glass of water.

## 6. Peppermint

Its menthol content will have a calming effect on the body.

Menthol is found in the peppermint herb.

Pain, inflammation, heartburn, swollen joints, diarrhea, dry mouth, and other symptoms are lessened by this herb's anti-inflammatory, digestive, and carminative properties.

Patients with scleroderma benefit from this herb in a natural and efficient manner.

## In what way

Early in the morning, on an empty stomach, take some fresh peppermint leaves and chew them.

Six to ten peppermint leaves in two cups of water can be used to make a herbal tea.

Drink this herbal tea once or twice a day by boiling it until there is only a half-cup left, straining the mixture as it cools. It is the best natural treatment for people with scleroderma.

## 7. Cinnamon

The herb cinnamon exhibits anti-oxidant, anti-inflammatory, and immuno-modulator properties. The active ingredient in cinnamon is cinnamonaldehyde.

## What to do

Take two cups of water and a stick of cinnamon herb. Boil this until there is one cup left, then strain the mixture to get the last cup. Use this herbal tea once or twice daily.

A teaspoon of ground cinnamon can also be dissolved in a glass of water. Boil this until remaining half, strain the mixture. Drink this herbal decoction once daily.

Use one of the aforementioned home remedies to naturally treat scleroderma.

## Best Way to Treat Scleroderma

CREST Syndrome is a form of scleroderma, a disease which stems from the overproduction and accumulation of collagen, a connective tissue protein. Scleroderma is an autoimmune disorder in which, for unknown reasons, the immune system attacks parts of the body's own circulatory system, leading to fibrosis and scarring. It primarily affects tiny blood vessels and can develop in almost any organ.

You can be diagnosed with CREST Syndrome if you have any two of the following five symptoms of this particular form of scleroderma:

**Calcinosis:** The formation of tiny deposits of calcium on the skin. These look like little hard white areas, usually on the elbows, knees or fingers.

**Raynaud's disease:** The spasm of tiny blood vessels in the fingers, toes, nose, tongue or ears upon exposure to very cold (or hot) temperatures or (sometimes) in response to stress. The affected areas turn white or bluish and may be painful.

**Esophageal disease:** A malfunctioning of the muscle of the lower part of the esophagus, which then allows stomach acid to flow back into the esophagus, causing heartburn and inflammation. This can result in scarring and may interfere with swallowing food.

**Sclerodactyly:** A thickening and tightness of the skin on the fingers or toes that limits motion.

**Telangiectasia:** The development of spidery, red patches on the face, hands, and in the mouth, due to abnormal proliferation of tiny blood vessels.

You might look into Chinese medicine for treatment of CREST Syndrome. I also would recommend taking the anti-inflammatory herbs ginger and turmeric as well as adopting an anti-inflammatory, plant-based diet with an emphasis on omega-3 fatty acids in the form of cold-water fish, fortified eggs, walnuts and flax.

You may also consider taking a fish oil supplement.

## How stress management can benefit those with chronic illness

Chronic stress can lead to many physical and emotional issues, such as anxiety, high blood pressure, stomach ulcers, and heart attacks. For many people with autoimmune diseases, stress causes a ton of complications and exacerbates symptoms.

This is also true for those of us with scleroderma, as stress can result in a Raynaud's phenomenon flare-up, heart palpitations, anxiety, or stomach issues. Mostly, it makes the painful symptoms we already endure worse, and it might even cause new issues to arise.

## The stress of scleroderma

We have to worry about eating right, getting enough sleep, and taking our prescribed medicine at the correct time and in the correct amount. Then there's the task of getting transportation to and from doctor appointments and making sure we arrive at the right time.

Next, we must wear the proper clothing, depending on the weather. If it's cold, layers it is. If it's windy or raining, snowing or hailing, wearing the right items when venturing outside is key to protecting our body and avoiding catching a virus or developing pneumonia. This is just a taste of what people with systemic scleroderma must worry about when leaving the house. These herbs are beneficial for relieving the signs & symptoms related to scleroderma patients.

Since many people must adhere to strict dietary guidelines, eating is a whole other dragon to slay. Making sure all of your fruits and vegetables are organic, avoiding chocolate or other caffeinated foods due to a heart condition, and worrying about your cereal being gluten-free can be stressful. The long list of dos and don'ts can be stressful or even seriously detrimental to one's health.

Living with a chronic illness can come with a confusing set of rules, which many people don't seem to comprehend. If following those rules while attempting to live a normal life doesn't stress us out, I don't know what does!

## Relieving everyday stress

I go through a wide range of feelings and pain every day as a result of scleroderma. But everyone manages stress, even though it manifests differently in healthy people.

Nobody can realistically or successfully live a completely stress-free life.

Therefore, there is no way for those of us with scleroderma to avoid stress: we can't.

We can, however, be mindful of reducing stress and finding healthy ways to let go of any negative emotions. This, in my opinion, is the most effective way to eradicate the stress bug from daily life.

Carmella, Amy's orange, white, and black cat, lies on a colorful quilt while gazing up at the camera.

Cat Carmella unwinds and encourages Amy to follow suit. Amy Gietzen took the picture.

There are many ways to reduce stress. You could practice yoga, meditate, or join a class or group that specializes in baking, drawing, gardening, or sewing. Having pets can be very advantageous to some people. I can unwind and unwind with the help of my three adorable and lovable fur babies. Along with quilting, painting, and reading, music is one of my favorite ways to decompress.

The important thing is to do whatever brings you joy and helps you let go of the "junk.". Relationships, general emotional and physical health, and stress management are all greatly improved by it.

We all benefit from letting go of our negative baggage.

## Do Long-Term Stress Lead to My Scleroderma?

I wouldn't wish scleroderma—the disease that keeps giving—on anyone. Would it be possible for me to exchange it for a gift card or an in-store credit?

Unfortunately, scleroderma does not offer a return policy. The moment you possess something, you are compelled to wear it, just like when Grandma gave you that hideous sweater for Christmas.

## I Must Make Room for Healing During Stressful Times

But no one really knows where it came from and how I got it, and I find that very intriguing. I'll get into my private eye mode and start looking into the matter.

Patients with scleroderma are experts at analyzing, learning, and investigating.

We examine every detail.

We'll discover the solutions.

The problem is that none of us can pinpoint a specific cause for having scleroderma. There are a variety of theories, but stress is my favorite.

We are all aware of the potential for stress in life and how it can impact us. Killer is stress. Being in a constant state of fight-or-flight causes an acute stress response, which maintains our body in its heightened state.

The term "homeostasis," which refers to a balanced state, is one that our bodies strive to maintain. Stress over a long period of time will wear down the body. A homeostatic imbalance has been linked to disease, according to scientific research.

I've been under moderate to extreme stress for the majority of my adult life. My capacity to compartmentalize my emotions is exceptional. I take care of anything that needs to be handled. The fact that you can manage it all doesn't imply that it isn't difficult.

Stress management presents a challenge for many of us. We might have families to support, careers to advance, and a plethora of other duties that are incumbent upon us. We can't afford to let the pressure get to us. And on top of everything else, those of us with scleroderma have to deal with a rare disease.

Scleroderma affects more women than men, though, by a factor of four. I believe there is a stereotype that stresses women out more. Our culture exhorts us to do and have everything. Even just that amount of pressure is extremely stressful.

Once we have scleroderma or another autoimmune disease, stress has a significant impact on the disease's severity and can cause flare-ups. So it makes sense that stress could cause an autoimmune reaction. When our body is under stress, every organ is affected.

The exact cause of my scleroderma is unknown to medical professionals. Now, all that matters is controlling my symptoms and, most importantly, halting the spread of the disease. I have to calm down in order to accomplish that.

Do whatever it takes to reduce stress if you or someone you know has scleroderma. I adore doing hot yoga. I find that the moist heat is very cleansing and that it helps my joints. Prior to beginning any exercise program, make sure to get your doctor's approval. Alternatively, you could do whatever makes you happy, including reading, writing, and creating.

## Preventing complications and lowering mortality in scleroderma

Some of the symptoms and signs of SSc may be reduced by lifestyle changes. Interventions for Raynaud's, such as keeping warm and shielding fingers and toes from injury and extreme cold, may stop damage. Vitamin C dosages above 1000 mg per day should be avoided by patients because they promote the production of collagen and increase its deposition. Exercise and physical and/or occupational therapy are essential for preserving mobility and reducing contractures. Smaller, more frequent meals may be necessary for patients with GI involvement rather than more substantial ones. Patients with SSc must keep their digital ulcers dry and clean and stay away from potentially corrosive and abrasive substances on their skin. 1,10.

## Therapeutic Management

Ideally, patients with SSc require ongoing, individualized care from a rheumatologist, particularly if dcSSc and visceral organ involvement manifest. Although there aren't any FDA-approved treatments specifically for SSc, the therapeutic goals of preventing complications and lowering morbidity can frequently be achieved with pharmacologic treatment.

## Treatment for Symptoms

Topical moisturizers ought to be used by all SSc patients.

Scleroderma of the scalp and forehead may be treated with topical corticosteroids, such as triamcinolone, to slow its progression and improve its symptoms. Histamine1 or histamine2 blockers, tricyclic antidepressants, and/or trazodone may be useful in the treatment of pruritus.

The first-line treatment for SSc-related digital vasculopathy is to use dihydropyridine calcium channel blockers (typically oral nifedipine). Patients who suffer from severe Raynaud's phenomenon or active digital ulcers may benefit from vasodilation using intravenous (IV) prostanoids, typically iloprost.

Bosentan is a medication that is being used for treating SSc more and more frequently. In patients who do not respond to treatment with calcium channel blockers and/or prostanoids, bosentan may lessen the frequency of new digital ulcers; however, it does not enhance healing. Patients with SSc-related pulmonary arterial hypertension (PAH) are also strongly advised to take the drug bosentan because studies show that it prolongs survival and preserves exercise capacity. In severe cases, IV epoprostenol may be used.

Sildenafil may also improve SSc-associated PAH.

Angiotensin-converting enzyme (ACE) inhibitors are renoprotective and effectively lower blood pressure in SSc patients if they experience SSc-associated renal crisis. ACE inhibitors shouldn't be prescribed as a preventative measure because they might lead to worse patient outcomes.

Gastroesophageal reflux, esophageal strictures, and proton pump inhibitors are all preventable. Taking laxatives might be necessary if constipation is a concern. Patients with symptoms of motility disturbances, such as dysphagia, may benefit from prokinetic medications (such as octreotide and cisapride). Due to bacterial overgrowth, some SSc patients experience malabsorption; experts advise rotating antibiotics for these patients.

## Taking care of the Pathology That Is Underlying

Common treatments include corticosteroids, which have immunosuppressive and anti-inflammatory effects. In order to prevent long-term side effects like osteoporosis, abnormalities in blood sugar levels, ocular disorders, and weight gain, oral prednisone may be used to treat arthralgias and myalgias for brief periods of time. Prednisone in doses greater than 40 mg daily is linked to an increased risk of scleroderma renal crisis;

alternative analgesics, such as nonsteroidal anti-inflammatory drugs and acetaminophen, are preferred if they work.

The differentiation and proliferation of keratinocytes are influenced by vitamin D analogues, such as oral calcitriol and topical calcipotriene ointment19. After 3 to 7 months of treatment, increased joint mobility and skin extensibility are the result of calcitriol's ability to inhibit fibroblast proliferation, collagen synthesis, and perhaps T-lymphocyte activation.

Immunosuppressants have also been used to treat SSc, with varying degrees of success. Clinicians have discussed the use of methotrexate with or without concurrent corticosteroids: a significant benefit was observed in treating resistant and active lcSSc, with no serious adverse reactions

175

reported after 3 to 6 months of treatment. Skin induration and handgrip strength were found to be better at 6 months of treatment in one randomized, placebo-controlled, double-blind study of 29 SSc patients receiving weekly methotrexate injections. Complete blood count (CBC), platelet count, liver function, blood urea nitrogen concentration, creatinine level, and estimated glomerular filtration rate must all be closely monitored in patients taking methotrexate.

Researchers have found that the interleukin-2 (IL-2) level is increased in early SSc, indicating that the IL-2 antagonist cyclosporine might be beneficial. According to small studies, cyclosporine reduces skin induration but has no impact on pulmonary or cardiac involvement. Use of it is constrained due to the risk of nephrotoxicity, especially at high doses (>3 mg/kg/day). Significant drug interactions exist with cyclosporine, and it also needs to be monitored for hypertension and bone marrow suppression. Mycophenolate mofetil may be a promising replacement for cyclophosphamide, according to recent studies.

## Antifibrotic Drugs

Collagen cross-linkages are impacted by the antifibrotic chelating agent D-penicillamine. After 38 months of follow-up, an early study found a significantly higher 5-year cumulative survival rate, a significantly reduced rate of new visceral organ involvement, and an improved degree and extent of skin thickness. In a later multicenter, double-blind, randomized clinical trial, it was discovered that using more than 125 mg every other day produced significantly more adverse events, such as proteinuria, but no additional improvement.

Colchicine may interfere with the synthesis of collagen, lessen the proliferation of fibroblasts, stimulate collagenase activity, and lessen inflammation. Colchicine appears to enhance skin elasticity, mouth opening, finger motility, and dysphagia and is typically well tolerated. A CBC as well as liver and renal function tests are included in monitoring.

Serious and intricate complications are common in SSc patients. For these patients, who frequently take a variety of medications, pharmacists' drug expertise is essential. Pharmacists may find it difficult to check patients for drug interactions and to explain the risks and benefits of various medications to patients. Patients must be closely watched for unfavorable events.